# Partnering *with* Caregivers

# Partnering *with* Caregivers

Learn How to Help Those Who Help Others

Verna Foster Harvey

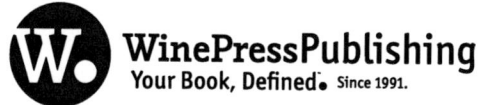

© 2010 by Verna Foster Harvey. All rights reserved.

WinePress Publishing (PO Box 428, Enumclaw, WA 98022) functions only as book publisher. As such, the ultimate design, content, editorial accuracy, and views expressed or implied in this work are those of the author.

No part of this publication may be reproduced, stored in a retrieval system, or transmitted in any way by any means—electronic, mechanical, photocopy, recording, or otherwise—without the prior permission of the copyright holder, except as provided by USA copyright law.

Unless otherwise noted, all Scriptures are taken from the *King James Version* of the Bible.

ISBN 13: 978-1-4141-1866-6
ISBN 10: 1-4141-1866-X
Library of Congress Catalog Card Number: 2010909332

## Disclaimer

This book is designed to provide information. It is not designed to dictate to anyone a particular course of action for any situation. The author shall have neither liability nor responsibility to any person or entity with respect to any loss or damage caused, or alleged to have been caused, directly or indirectly, by the information contained in this book. *If you do not wish to be bound by the above, you may return this book to the publisher for a full refund.*

# Contents

An Appeal of Assistance . . . . . . . . . . . . . . . . . . . . . . . . . . . . . .ix
Appreciation . . . . . . . . . . . . . . . . . . . . . . . . . . . . . . . . . . . . . .xi
Foreword. . . . . . . . . . . . . . . . . . . . . . . . . . . . . . . . . . . . . . . .xiii
Introduction: A Brief Chronological Snapshot of How
    I Became a Caregiver . . . . . . . . . . . . . . . . . . . . . . . . . . . xv

1. Establishing the Foundation: Who Should
    Read This Book?. . . . . . . . . . . . . . . . . . . . . . . . . . . . . . . . 1
2. Who is This Coordinator?. . . . . . . . . . . . . . . . . . . . . . . . . . 2
3. Is a Caregiver Coordinator Really Necessary? . . . . . . . . . . 3
4. When is the Ministry Needed? . . . . . . . . . . . . . . . . . . . . . . 4
5. How Caregivers are Chosen . . . . . . . . . . . . . . . . . . . . . . . . 5
6. The Responsibilities of the Caregiver . . . . . . . . . . . . . . . . . 6
7. Additional Responsibilities of the Caregiver:
    Patient's Need of Special Services. . . . . . . . . . . . . . . . . . 8
8. Immediate Needs: When the Patient Goes Home. . . . . . . . 9
9. Duties Designated "For Caregivers Only". . . . . . . . . . . . . 11
10. Understanding the Ministry of
    the Caregiver's Coordinator . . . . . . . . . . . . . . . . . . . . . 13
11. Helpers: How They Contribute. . . . . . . . . . . . . . . . . . . . 15
12. The Caregiver's Coordinator: Is this Role Biblical? . . . . . . . 17

13. The Coordinator's Oath of Responsibility. . . . . . . . . . . . . . 19
14. Should Family Members be Appointed
    as Coordinators?. . . . . . . . . . . . . . . . . . . . . . . . . . . . . . . . 20
15. Who Should be Appointed as Coordinator?. . . . . . . . . . . 21
16. Who Will Help Mobile Families to Receive Assistance?. . . 22
17. Should an Alternate Coordinator be Appointed?. . . . . . . . . 23
18. Managing Negative Responses . . . . . . . . . . . . . . . . . . . . . 24
19. Caregiver's Basic Instructions to the Coordinator. . . . . . . . 26
20. Establishing Communication Lists. . . . . . . . . . . . . . . . . . 27
21. Communication: The Inner Circle . . . . . . . . . . . . . . . . . 28
22. Other Communication Lists . . . . . . . . . . . . . . . . . . . . . . 30
23. Appointing Prayer Warriors . . . . . . . . . . . . . . . . . . . . . . 32
24. Communicating via the Internet (Web sites) or E-mail . . . 33
25. Using Facebook as a Means of Communication. . . . . . . . 35
26. Alternative Care Pages: Free Web sites . . . . . . . . . . . . . . . 36
27. Can Men Function as Coordinators? . . . . . . . . . . . . . . . . 37
28. Sending Flowers to the Patient . . . . . . . . . . . . . . . . . . . . 38
29. Helping Out-of-Towners to Lend a Helping Hand . . . . . . . . . 40
30. Other Suggestions for Out-of-Towners . . . . . . . . . . . . . . . 42
31. Miscellaneous Services the Patient Will Need at Home . . . 43
32. Types of Services the Patient *Does Not* Need! . . . . . . . . . . 45
33. The Patient and Caregiver's New Way of Life. . . . . . . . . . 47
34. When Should Hospice be Considered?. . . . . . . . . . . . . . . 49
35. Give the Caregiver Plenty of Breaks!. . . . . . . . . . . . . . . . . 50
36. Encourage the Caregiver to Seek Support from
    Other Caregivers. . . . . . . . . . . . . . . . . . . . . . . . . . . . . . . 54
37. Calling Partners/Agencies for Assistance . . . . . . . . . . . . . 56
38. Caring for the Children in the Family . . . . . . . . . . . . . . . 58
39. Arrange Fun Time for the Children—Give
    Them a Break!. . . . . . . . . . . . . . . . . . . . . . . . . . . . . . . . 61
40. Family Matters . . . . . . . . . . . . . . . . . . . . . . . . . . . . . . . 62

Conclusion . . . . . . . . . . . . . . . . . . . . . . . . . . . . . . . . . . . . . 63
About the Author . . . . . . . . . . . . . . . . . . . . . . . . . . . . . . . . 65

# An Appeal of Assistance

As we have therefore opportunity, let us do good unto all men, especially unto them who are of the household of faith.
—Galatians 6:10

BELOVED, USING THE information provided in this book, it is my hope and prayer that you will partner with a caregiver to assist him or her in at least one of the many practical ways outlined. Each of our journeys here on this earth is a distinct one; however, the voyage is more tolerable and enjoyable when someone is on the same path with us. Won't you please help to lighten the burdens of just one individual?

Affectionately yours,
**Verna**

# Appreciation

RECORDED IN THIS book are some of the lessons I learned while being a caregiver to my husband. Without the trial, I would not have obtained this personal knowledge. I pray the outcome of both, the book and the trial, glorifies my Father in heaven, whom I worship and follow.

I really, really, really appreciate you, Lenon Harvey, my husband and best friend, for your contribution to this book project and to my life. The love, wisdom, and guidance you provide is always needed and appreciated. I can never say enough about the support you give me every time I embark on another project. This support alone is priceless.

Foster Harvey, our youngest child (and my personal, in-house editor!), thank you for tirelessly reading almost everything I have written. I also thank you for your great insight and for letting me know when something that I write really touches you. I will miss your many contributions when you leave home for college next year!

Jacinta Harvey, our daughter, thank you for providing the Foreword to this book. I especially thank you for making life a little easier for me during the time of your dad's surgery and recuperation. Your assistance will not be forgotten.

L.C., our eldest son; Mandy, his wife; and Mikade, Mikah, and Noah, their children—you bring us much joy!

Troy Thomas Jr., our godson, you are growing up to be quite a gentleman. Thank you for always remembering those special occasions. You are very dear to our hearts.

My youngest sister, Anita Ozell Foster, thank you for arranging the benefit program, Under the Overflow, held at Fifth Street Baptist Church in Meridian, Mississippi, on our behalf during a very dark time in our lives. Our sincere thanks also go to the overseer, Bishop William C. Brown, and the leaders and members at Fifth Street for your willingness to host this event. Finally, thank you to our family members and friends who assisted with this program.

Pastor Luther Barnes and the Redd Bud Gospel Choir, thank you so very, very much for your contribution to help make the benefit program a success. This priceless gift to us was a blessing sent by God, through you, to my family. I will always remember how your loving kindness touched my family's hearts.

Family members, friends, churches near and far, thank you for your prayers, encouraging words, donated leave, monetary offerings, and all other acts of kindness. Your tender thoughts, especially during our crisis, will forever be a testimony of your love toward us. Your actions demonstrate the sentiments embodied in my favorite Bible verse, Psalm 40, verse 5:

> Many, oh LORD my God, are thy wonderful works which thou hast done, and thy thoughts which are to us-ward: they cannot be reckoned up in order unto thee: if I would declare and speak of them, they are more than can be numbered.

I cannot give an account by providing names for every person who provided assistance to my family; neither can I tally the blessings that overflowed from your heart to ours. All I know is that this journey was unique because it brought together people from around the world—many whom I have never had the pleasure of meeting. To every person who journeyed with us, I say, "Thank you. *To God Be the Glory.*"

A child of the King,
**Verna**

# Foreword

BEING A CAREGIVER is hard work. It takes a lot of patience, dedication, and perseverance. It's a task that at times can be very rewarding and at other times may seem like it is almost impossible, especially if you are carrying the load on your own.

As a therapist, one fact I find myself constantly having to remind my clients of is that in order to take care of others, they have to take care of their needs first. If you have ever flown and actually listened to the flight attendants' speech before the plane takes off, you may recall that they tell you to put your oxygen mask on yourself before you try to assist anybody else. Before you can help others, you first have to be in a position/condition to be able to give effective help. Therefore, caregivers must learn to take care of themselves.

With this in mind, caregivers must be open to the gift of helps that others are willing to give. Likewise, family members and friends (partners) of caregivers must be willing to extend that necessary hand of help. Partners of caregivers provide the loving support that is needed by efficiently tending to volunteered or delegated duties. This partnership empowers the caregiver and helps him or her perform his or her duty of care to the patient with ease. It is imperative to lift one another up when the need arises.

—Jacinta Y. Harvey, LAPC

# Introduction
## A Brief Chronological Snapshot of How I Became a Caregiver

THE INTRODUCTION YOU are about to read chronicles the events surrounding my husband's illness and the process we both endured in order to get to the point where we are now. When reading the forty short chapters that follow this introduction, try to place yourself in the path of a caregiver and see how you can help him or her. If there ever is a time that your service is needed, it is when a caregiver is in the midst of taking care of his or her loved one. Beloved, it is my prayer that the love in your heart will guide you to the hearts of those who need a helping hand. Moreover, where your heart leads you, I trust you will follow.

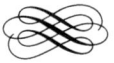

Many people who knew my husband, Len, prior to his surgery would find it hard to believe he was having medical problems. Len, a veteran of the armed services, was known for keeping himself fit. His physique highlighted the fact that he frequently worked out at a local gym. He was the picture of health. In fact, even when he was hospitalized before his surgery, doctors and nurses would constantly say to him, "You don't look like you're sick." Well, I can assure you, it is possible for a person to be seriously ill and yet not look sick.

Len suffered many months with frequent nausea, dizziness, and hearing loss. Although the symptoms may not seem severe, they were aggravating enough to keep him from working his normal schedule. For this combination of problems, Len sought the advice of many different doctors. Every time he saw a new doctor, a different test would be conducted, resulting in a new diagnosis. Yet none of the medicines prescribed ever remedied any of the problems. Then, one day, Len's temporary primary care provider asked him to walk heel-to-toe. Immediately upon Len's failing this test, an MRI of the brain was ordered. This test was completed on October 18, 2007.

On Wednesday morning, October 31, Len went back to the clinic for a follow-up appointment. However, this time he was scheduled to see someone other than his temporary primary care provider. This treating physician was on a temporary duty assignment from a base in Texas. The follow-up exam was completed, and the doctor assumed that everything was normal with Len's MRI since the results were not in his medical records. She also indicated that had there been a concern, his physician would have been notified. Nevertheless, this God-sent angel followed up on Len's inquiry regarding the results of the MRI.

Near 3:30 in the afternoon, Len was notified by telephone that the military physician, whom he had seen that morning, wanted to see us in her office ASAP. Once I was notified, I immediately informed my supervisor and left work. My drive from work to the base was calm, much like the quietness often experienced before a storm.

Once we were in the doctor's office, the physician looked at Len and said, "I know you are a godly man. One reason I know this is because when I saw you this morning, you were reading your Bible. And after I began to speak with you, I could really tell." She went on to say, "The moment I received your MRI results, I started praying." She then began to explain the purpose of our visit, while simultaneously handing us a copy of the MRI report. The first

## A Brief Chronological Snapshot of How I Became a Caregiver

words on the report under the Findings section was, *Examination is markedly abnormal.* What followed was a detailed description of the tumor that was detected. The tumor's size was 4.7 centimeters by 4.2 centimeters, which is approximately 1 ½ inches by 1 ¼ inches. Other than the size, only speculative information was included. Further analysis would take place at a later date.

The discovery of the tumor was shocking, and it warranted our concern. I also was troubled about not being notified sooner of the findings. I felt that there was absolutely no reason for the lengthy delay! Whether the communication problem was at the site where the MRI was performed or internally at the base, I do not know. What I do know is that this visiting physician had to request a copy of the report from the facility where the test was performed in order for the documentation to be put in Len's records and for us to be told of the findings. Had the physician not requested a copy, who knows if we ever would have found out about the tumor before irreparable damage occurred.

At this point, I did indicate to the physician that this delay in communication needed addressing. She assured me, the matter had already been brought to the attention of those in command. Since I had other, more important matters to deal with, I did not inquire any further into the incident. I felt assured that this physician would handle the matter in the appropriate manner. My purpose in having the matter addressed was to prevent what happened to us from occurring to anyone else.

With my focus now on Len, the doctor informed us that once she received the MRI results, she started making telephone calls to secure an appointment with a neurologist in another city. Nearly everything needed was in place except an exact date and time when Len would be admitted to the hospital for further testing. The doctor assured us that the moment this information was communicated to her, she would notify us.

Meanwhile, after we left the doctor's office, we discussed how we should tell our children. Since our eldest son would be visiting us for the weekend, we decided to wait until Saturday, especially considering the fact that our youngest child Foster's birthday was on Friday. We certainly wanted Foster to enjoy *his day* without having to think about his dad's illness.

I went to bed that night with a heavy heart. Not having a definite course of action in place and not knowing when the process would start was difficult. All we could do at this point was to pray and wait.

The next morning, we started the day out by following our normal routine. Len left home for work, Foster left for school, and then I left for work. Yet, Thursday, November 1, 2007, will be the one day of my life I will always remember. Not long after we reached our destinations, Len received a telephone call from the doctor who performed the follow-up exam. He was told to report to a hospital in Augusta, Georgia, which is about 250 miles away, to see a neurologist ASAP. Because time was of the essence, I choose to stay behind and take care of Foster while a military friend drove Len to the hospital.

After this arrangement was made, I then realized our original plan to tell the children about the illness on Saturday was not feasible. Because of Len's leaving so suddenly, and the fact that he would not be returning home, I was left with no choice but to tell the children prior to Foster's birthday. This difficult task had to be done without their father, my husband, being nearby to comfort them and encourage me. My heart pondered on this throughout the majority of the day.

If ever there was an inopportune time for an illness to occur, this was it. We had such busy schedules. Len worked full time, when he wasn't sick from the tumor. I worked a full-time job as a paralegal and part-time as an instructor. Foster was involved in school sports. We were very active in our church, always doing what we could when we could. Yet I knew God had a purpose for what was going on in our lives. But with the process just beginning, I did not have the slightest idea what He was doing and how long this trial would last. Neither did I know the amount of pain that would accompany this trial.

As I thought about how I would tell the children of their dad's illness, I knew my only way of informing our eldest son, L.C., was

## A Brief Chronological Snapshot of How I Became a Caregiver

via telephone. Therefore, I concentrated more on how to go about telling the two children at home. In fact, a telephone call was made to L.C. later that day. In our conversation, I also informed him that I would be telling his sister and brother later that night. With this being said, he knew not to say anything to them until after we talked again.

Since our daughter, Jacinta, did not live with us, I had to arrange for her to pick up Foster once he returned home from school and after her college classes ended. I wanted Foster to be with his sister so that he would not be inquiring about his dad not being at home. It turned out, Jacinta had a tutoring session scheduled, so I arranged for Foster to join her while she was tutoring. Then, once I finished teaching, I picked Foster up and went home to wait for Jacinta to join us.

Once we were all home, I explained to Jacinta and Foster what the doctor had shared with their dad and me and where he was. We embraced one another and cried. They both took the announcement really hard, especially Jacinta. I knew that because she was a graduate student studying psychology, she had a greater understanding of the brain, and the typical outcome for most patients. At this time, I had to remind her that book knowledge is good, but she should not underestimate the power of God. I told her to leave space in her heart for God to work a miracle in every patient.

Later that night, Len called home. The sound of his voice provided some relief for the children. However, the process was just beginning, and we still had no answers.

The hospital performed tests throughout the night on Len. Through their testing, we found out that the tumor was benign. Praise God! This news was comforting, but the epidermoid tumor needed to be removed. Surgery was scheduled for November 14. In the meantime, Len's doctor told him he could not drive, do any strenuous activities, or return to work until after the surgery. With this news, I began to wonder how we would survive, since nearly all of his sick leave had been exhausted. Not to mention the fact that we did not have a clue as to how long after the surgery he would need in order to heal. My heart searched for answers that were not readily available.

After I arrived home from work on Friday, November 2 (Foster's birthday), the children and I drove to Augusta to pick up Len. We were weary from the journey, but delighted to be back together again. Foster's birthday wasn't as cheerful as we had hoped for, but we did the best we could, considering the circumstances.

We still did not know exactly what to expect, and the days ahead were rough. It was as if we were waiting for a time bomb to explode.

Prior to the surgery, I remember waking up very early one morning. Being led by God, I sent an e-mail to nearly every person in my e-mail address book, soliciting prayer and help for our situation. My main purpose was to ask for contributions of donated leave for Len. I knew of this leave-donation program because I had contributed to someone in need when I was a federal government employee. Now, since Len was a federal employee and I knew we needed help, I was led by God to ask for assistance from others. This was a humbling experience, but it generated responses from people locally as well as in other states, most of whom I didn't even know, because the e-mail was forwarded several times. Although the mandatory procedure used to process the leave was complex, once all requirements were met, the help we received was invaluable. (Len was also able to use advanced sick leave.) With these two systems in place, my mind was relieved of one huge burden.

Len's surgery was performed on Wednesday, November 14, at the Medical College of Georgia (MCG). A few members of our former church, including the pastor and his wife, met us at the hospital that morning to pray with us prior to the surgery. Even though the surgery lasted about eight hours, most of the members stayed with me while the surgery was being performed. According to the doctors, everything went well. However, due to the fact that the tumor was located near the brain stem, only 85% of it could be removed safely. The remaining 15% will be monitored throughout the remainder of Len's life. Additionally, because the tumor was not cancerous, the residual could not be treated with radiation or chemotherapy; for now, it's just a thorn that keeps us both before the Lord.

## A Brief Chronological Snapshot of How I Became a Caregiver

The doctors decided Len was well enough to leave the hospital on Monday, November 19. But after being home for a short while, Len started having problems. On Sunday, November 25, a little before midnight, I telephoned the doctor in Augusta and made him aware of the severe headache Len was experiencing. I was told to take him to the Emergency Room for further diagnosis. Since we were a great distance from Augusta, I took Len to the Emergency Room at a nearby hospital. After being examined, Len was admitted to the hospital. Based on the symptoms he was experiencing—fever, stiffness around the neck area, and other closely-related symptoms—doctors thought he had meningitis. Different tests ruled out this and other similar illnesses. Once Len was stabilized, the doctors decided it was best for him to be treated by the physician who performed his surgery. After arrangements were made, on Wednesday, November 28, Len was transported by ambulance to MCG, where he only spent a few days in the hospital. On Saturday, December 1, the children and I traveled to Augusta to pick him up from the hospital and bring him home.

On Sunday, December 9, right before breakfast, I noticed a clear fluid leaking out of the surgically-stitched area on Len's head. After receiving permission from our insurance company, Len was taken to the Emergency Room at MCG. I opted not to take him to a local hospital, given the fact that the last time he was seen, he was transported back to the doctor who performed the surgery. Doctors are very cautious about treating patients who have had brain surgery. We have found out they prefer that the surgical doctor treat his or her own patients because the risk to them is so great.

The doctor who examined Len in the Emergency Room at MCG did not see what I saw. Needless to say, we returned home without the assurance of knowing that everything was OK. (This doctor later recognized his misdiagnosis and asked us openly for forgiveness. Because of this acknowledgement, we knew he had made an honest mistake. At that moment, we began to pray continuously for him. We knew in our hearts that one day he would be a great physician, because humbleness was one of the medicines he provided to patients.)

Just two days later, on Tuesday, December 11, Len had a regularly scheduled follow-up appointment at MCG. The nurse practitioner who examined Len's wound immediately notified doctors of the leakage she saw, and once again, Len was admitted to the hospital. This time he needed a lumbar drain in order to remove some of the cerebrospinal fluid that was leaking from his head and to regulate the flow inside his brain and spine. Throughout this process, Len had continuous headaches, and occasional nausea developed. The headaches were controlled with medication, but the nausea lingered on for days.

Len was finally dismissed from the hospital on Friday, December 21, just in time to be home for Christmas. This holiday was different. Although we were home, it was a very challenging time for us. While home, Len could not keep food in his stomach. His doctor thought the nausea would eventually subside, but it did not. Len was given different types of medications, but nothing worked perfectly. Meanwhile, he continued to lose weight.

On Thursday, January 3, 2008, by the time we arrived for Len's scheduled follow-up appointment at MCG, his doctor had decided Len needed to be admitted to the hospital. During this stay, Len was treated primarily for dehydration.

On Saturday, January 5, Len was dismissed from the hospital. When he came home this time, he finally started gaining some of his strength back. However, somewhere in the midst of being sick, his voice became hoarse and never returned to normal. This new problem necessitated a referral to an ear, nose, and throat specialist. Visits to this specialist eventually yielded that surgery was necessary in order to correct the problem he was experiencing.

In the meantime, Len continued to heal, and with the doctor's permission, he decided to return to work part time, with limited duties. Working part time was quite a struggle, but Len insisted. Then near the end of May, he started working full time.

This throat surgery that Len needed was scheduled to be performed at a local hospital on Monday, June 9. Well, the surgery actually never took place because the doctor stated that when Len was positioned for the doctor to perform the necessary procedure,

## A Brief Chronological Snapshot of How I Became a Caregiver

there was nothing to repair; the problem had corrected itself! Len's voice did improve, and we celebrated this milestone with great joy.

Everything appeared to be going well, until Monday, June 30. On this morning, I received an e-mail from Len while he was at work. The e-mail stated, "Hi, Babe, I don't know what's wrong with me, I just feel sick all over my body. Please pray my strength in the Lord." It wasn't long after I received this message that he telephoned me at work, stating that he did not feel well and I needed to come pick him up. I immediately left work.

When I arrived at the shop where he worked, he could barely walk outside. It was apparent that something was terribly wrong. Since Len worked on base, I took him to the clinic, hoping he could see a doctor to get some type of medicine to ease the severe pain in his head. I did inform the doctors of Len's previous surgery, but they thought perhaps he was having a migraine because of the symptoms he displayed. While the doctors at the base were treating Len, I telephoned his doctor at MCG and explained the situation. His doctor advised me to bring Len to the hospital in the morning.

When we arrived at the hospital Tuesday morning, July 1, a MRI was performed. The image on the MRI showed that a cyst containing fluid had formed in the area where the tumor had been removed. This build-up of fluid was causing extreme pressure, which was responsible for the headache Len was experiencing. Len was admitted to the hospital, and surgery to remove the cyst was performed the very next day, July 2. The surgery went well, and again, Len was on the road to recovery.

Prior to being dismissed from the hospital on Friday, July 4, Len asked his doctor if he could attend his brother's funeral in another state. (Len's brother died June 27, and his funeral was on July 5.) The doctor very solemnly indicated to us that it was best for Len to go straight home and rest.

For the next few months, we took frequent trips to Augusta for doctors' appointments at MCG. All of the visits indicated that Len was continuing to heal, but he still had frequent headaches, and the problem with his voice reoccurred.

Eventually, Len was referred to a specialist at MCG for his voice. This doctor stated that as a result of the surgeries and perhaps the complications experienced, Len had a paralyzed vocal cord and would need surgery in order for it to be repaired. Outpatient surgery was performed at MCG on Thursday, January 29, 2009.

Throughout the healing process, Len has had continuous physical therapy. He has had speech therapy for about eighteen months. Although things in our lives are relatively stable, nothing exists the way it did before this illness occurred. We have learned that Len's medical condition dictates his activities, and it affects ours. Sometimes Len has extremely good days, and sometimes his days are spent nursing his many ailments. During these times, more of the household responsibilities fall on me. You know, that's perfectly OK, because through this illness, I have learned that dust is not my highest priority! As Jesus told Martha, "…one thing is needful…" (Luke 10:42), and I am happy to say that I have chosen that good part—God first and then my family.

# Chapter 1
## Establishing the Foundation: Who Should Read This Book?

THIS BOOK IS *not* for the patient. It is written with the caregiver in mind, but it is not intended to be used primarily by the caregiver. (Although, during a crisis, it may be beneficial to the caregiver as a guide.) Rather, this book is intended for those who partner with caregivers. A partner can be anyone who desires to lend a helping hand to a family member, friend, coworker, neighbor, stranger, etc., who is facing a crisis. This person could be *you*!

Partners are needed to assist with the many responsibilities caregivers endure. However, when multiple hands are involved in an activity, one person needs to coordinate the services that are provided. The person who oversees the administration of the care provided to assist caregivers is affectionately called a "caregiver coordinator." This term is used throughout this book and will be further defined in the next chapter.

# Chapter 2
## Who is This Coordinator?

IN GENERAL, A coordinator is the person responsible for planning an event. In this case, the caregiver coordinator helps to organize and/or harmonize the services a patient and caregiver receive, thus reducing the responsibilities of the caregiver.

Wait! Before this book is tossed aside, be comforted in knowing that this ministry will not last a lifetime. It is designed to:

1. Help meet immediate needs by establishing a helpline of support for the patient and caregiver.
2. Assist the caregiver in adjusting to a new way of life.
3. Help ease the transferring of responsibilities back to the caregiver once a crisis has stabilized or the situation has returned to normal.

# Chapter 3
# Is a Caregiver Coordinator Really Necessary?

NOT ALL SITUATIONS will warrant the services of a coordinator. However, in those cases in which coordinators are needed, they are truly needed and appreciated! Just to get a general idea of the service coordinators provide, imagine planning for a big event, such as a wedding, a family reunion, or perhaps a big formal gathering, without any assistance from anyone. Imagine being the only person making all the decisions surrounding the event. (Are you screaming for help yet?) Caregivers, for the most part, are in a similar position. This is why they need someone, a coordinator, to partner with them by helping to manage the new and demanding responsibilities that suddenly surfaced in their lives. Coordinators can help to prevent the burnout most caregivers encounter after a tragedy has occurred. Remember, tragedies are not planned; they normally happen without any advance warning. A tragedy could happen to anyone, including you.

# Chapter 4

# When is the Ministry Needed?

ONE OF THE most trying times for a family normally begins with the onset of a crisis. When a crisis occurs, the person closest to the patient is usually overwhelmed with the details of the situation and decisions that must be made about medical care. Instead of just saying to a caregiver, "Don't worry about this or that, you just focus on (the name of the patient or patients)," the activation of the coordinator ministry helps to put those words into action. The coordinator helps to relieve the caregiver of additional responsibilities, thereby releasing the caregiver's mind and enabling him or her to concentrate on the direct needs of the patient and on emotional needs as well.

# Chapter 5

# How Caregivers are Chosen

WHEN A MEDICAL mishap occurs, all decisions about medical care normally reside with the relative who is the nearest of kin. When the sick person is the husband, normally the wife has this responsibility, and vice versa when the wife is the patient. In situations involving children, parents sometimes make decisions jointly. However, when families are no longer intact, which is now the norm, decisions made on behalf of a child/children can become a battle ground. In other cases, siblings make decisions for either a parent or a sibling. No matter whom this decision-making person is, in most cases, this person ends up assuming the role of caregiver to the patient. In short, a caregiver doesn't always volunteer for the position; most are appointed because of their association to the patient. There also are times when a person may choose to take the position out of guilt.

## Chapter 6
## The Responsibilities of the Caregiver

C AREGIVERS' RESPONSIBILITIES ARE numerous and never-ending. Primarily, caregivers are responsible for the numerous medical decisions that must be made for the patient. This in itself is a tremendous responsibility! Not only is the caregiver receiving information from the medical staff, but also a concerned caregiver most often seeks additional information from other sources. Although the research process takes up valuable time, most caregivers will take whatever time is necessary in order to educate themselves about their loved one's illness. This research is done so that the caregiver, who hopefully is already equipped with spiritual knowledge, will be equipped with the best possible medical knowledge. A firm understanding of the illness and the choices available will enable the caregiver to make crucial decisions with a high level of assurance. Having the ability to make wise decisions is comforting.

Next, think about the countless hours caregivers spend at the bedside of a patient while he or she is in the hospital. Sometimes a patient can be taken care of in a nearby hospital, which makes adjusting to the situation a little easier. However, that's not always possible. My husband's surgery was performed in a city located over 250 miles away from our hometown. Therefore, I did not have the luxury of going home on a daily basis. My household chores and other responsibilities were put on hold, which meant that little by little, things at home began to get out of order. Unfortunately, displacement for caregivers is becoming more of the norm, especially when a crisis requires specialty services for a patient.

# Chapter 7
## Additional Responsibilities of the Caregiver: Patient's Need of Special Services

WHEN PATIENTS ARE not allowed to go directly home after they are discharged from the hospital, they oftentimes are admitted into a nursing home or a rehabilitation facility. This is done for various reasons. One is because patients must to be able to perform certain functions before doctors will allow them to go home. To assist patients in learning these functions, doctors transfer patients to some type of facility where these skills are taught. Another reason some patients do not go home is because no one is available to be with them on a continuous basis while they are home recuperating. Then there are other patients who cannot go home because although a person may be available to be with a patient, that person is not physically able to care for the patient. None of these scenarios totally dismisses a caregiver from his or her responsibilities. Instead, another layer of concern (stress) is added.

# Chapter 8
## Immediate Needs: When the Patient Goes Home

AFTER THE PATIENT is discharged from the hospital, nursing home, or other type of facility, then many responsibilities will fall directly on the caregiver. This is when help is most needed!

Some of the patient's immediate, day-to-day needs are listed below:

- Oversight of the administration of prescribed medicines
- Patient's hygiene (Heavy patients are more cumbersome to care for.)
- Preparation of foods (especially in cases where a special diet is prescribed)
- Recording daily vital signs
- Assistance/oversight when moving from place to place

Even with these few responsibilities (there are many more), no caregiver should bear the burden of caring for a patient all alone, as there are many other duties that must be handled directly by the caregiver. Look again at the above list. Which of these duties can be assigned to family members or friends?

After my husband was released from the hospital, recovering from brain tumor surgery, he could not sleep in a regular bed because his head needed to be elevated at about a fifty to sixty-degree angle; otherwise, he suffered from severe headaches. We tried using pillows and the wedge given to us at the hospital, but neither helped. The only other option I knew of at that time was for my husband to sleep in his recliner. This he did for the next six months. Because I needed to be by his side to assist him when he got up, I slept right beside him, on the couch. (He was very weak and could have fallen on the way to the bathroom or other areas of the house.) I would not have expected anyone else to take on this task, but there were other areas where help was needed, if only I would have allowed someone to assist me.

Minor tasks, such as the preparation of food, should be shifted from the caregiver to someone who is willing to help. (See chapter 31 for more suggestions.) There are always things designated "for caregiver only," so shifting minor things early in the crisis will help the caregiver in ways that cannot be imagined!

# Chapter 9
## Duties Designated "For Caregivers Only"

SOME OF THE duties that must be handled by the caregiver are listed below:

- Tending to personal financial obligations (Never suggest to a caregiver that this responsibility will be assumed by the coordinator or any helper!)
- Making doctors' appointments
- Communicating with doctors and/or nurses (except in cases of emergency)
- Filing for disability compensation (Timely filing is crucial. In most cases, the start date of disability is dependent upon when the paperwork was initiated, not when the disability first occurred.)

Handling any of the above matters, especially filing for disability compensation, consumes a lot of time! When the caregiver devotes attention to these important matters, other matters that need tending to are normally neglected. In my case, many things were neglected for an extremely long time. This, again, is where the coordinator can help to ensure that someone is taking care of other areas while the caregiver is focusing on more important tasks. (It's been over thirty months since my husband's first surgery, and my household is just beginning to get back to a state of normalcy. Praise the Lord!)

# Chapter 10
## Understanding the Ministry of the Caregiver's Coordinator

UNLESS YOU HAVE walked in the shoes of a caregiver, chances are you may know to do a few things that are helpful, but not as much as an experienced caregiver would know. One reason for this is that spectators have a different view; they are on the outside, looking in. But a person who has been totally involved in a crisis knows. Experience does make a difference.

For example, those who have never raised children can offer suggestions, but in nearly all cases, everyone knows the most valuable information about children can be obtained from a parent. And even parents know that their knowledge is limited because every child they come in contact with is different. Therefore, learning about a child is always a work in progress. Parenting doesn't come with a flip-chart, cure-all remedy!

When my three children were younger, disciplining the eldest child by restricting his phone usage wasn't effective because he didn't use the telephone that often. He lived in Germany for nearly nine years, where, due to the cost, telephone usage was extremely limited. But the younger two, especially my daughter, were quick to catch on to the good old American way! Telephone usage was essential to my daughter and quickly became a "can't-live-without" necessity for her. Therefore, when disciplining my children, I had to know what mattered the most and least to them; otherwise, my chastising would not have been effective.

Even though I managed to get through a very emotional and trying time in my life, speaking from the caregiver's perspective, the pains of my journey could have been lessened had someone partnered with me. A helper could have coordinated the assistance I most desperately needed. Honestly, I did not know I needed a variety of assistance at the time. Most caregivers do not. It wasn't until I was coming out of my crisis that I realized my mistake of not accepting help from those who offered.

This is where the coordinator's role is vital. Caregivers are overwhelmed at their initial appointment. They simply do not understand what their mission will entail. Furthermore, it's not like they were "expecting" a crisis the way parents "expect" a newborn baby. Circumstances are quite different for a caregiver. This is why all caregivers need someone to come alongside them to assist in the ministry they may have been thrust into. They need someone to help lift their burdens.

By having a coordinator in place, those general, sincere offers of, "If you need anything, please call," can quickly turn into commitments when the coordinator asks questions like, "Are you available to do grocery shopping, cut grass, sit with the patient for a short time, cook, send e-mails, pick up medications, pray, etc." With a coordinator in place, immediately, a schedule of care can be started and maintained. The establishment of this list allows family members and friends to partner in this ministry by lending a helping hand in *their* areas of expertise. Additionally, the coordinator is equipped with a list of helpers/partners and then easily can coordinate services as the caregiver desires and/or needs.

# Chapter II
## Helpers: How They Contribute

JUST A FEW years ago, I was one of a few on a coordinator's list. I assisted in providing care to a church member who had surgery and did not have any immediate family members in the area. I contributed by sitting with the patient in the hospital and at her home, driving her to doctors' appointments, and picking up medications from the pharmacy. Whatever the coordinator needed me to do for the patient, I did. Other female helpers assisted too. Most importantly, when help was needed from men, they gladly contributed as well. And the coordinator did all of the planning without even knowing she was functioning in this capacity!

When my husband was discharged from the hospital that was in another city, he would receive, like most patients, prescriptions for medications. Because our trip back to our hometown took nearly five hours, the medicine he received at the hospital prior to being discharged would start to wear off. Because of policy regulations, the hospital would not give us medicine to take with us. So on many occasions, I would call my daughter on the way home and have her meet us at a designated area just inside the city limits of the town where we lived. From that point, she would get her dad's prescriptions and take them to the nearest pharmacy to have them filled. Most times, the prescriptions were for controlled medicines, so they could not be called in or faxed to the pharmacy. Meanwhile, I was able to go home and start preparing a light meal or doing other necessary tasks.

Many months into our crisis, I was talking to a friend on my cell phone and explaining the situation to her. She suggested I get the prescriptions filled before leaving the area where I was. I explained to her that I could not locate a pharmacy in the area that accepted my insurance. This friend diligently searched the Internet until she found stores in the area that accepted my insurance. Using the Internet, she also provided a telephone number and directions to the stores. This partner's assistance was priceless! (Having a partner who knows how to use the Internet will be a great asset to any ministry.)

Caregivers must learn to make their needs known so that others who are removed from the situation can think for them and provide solutions to or make suggestions regarding the problem at hand. Fresh eyes have fresh insight. It's too late for me and my situation, but it is not for others and theirs.

# Chapter 12
## The Caregiver's Coordinator: Is this Role Biblical?

WHEN GOD CREATED Moses, He equipped him with everything needed to accomplish His will. However, Moses had to go through a process in order to develop the skill of using what was already given to him. Without the developmental process, Moses would not have matured as he did.

One weak area in Moses' life that did not develop to his own satisfaction was his voice. In Exodus 4:10, Moses told God, "…O my Lord, I am not eloquent, neither heretofore, nor since thou hast spoken unto thy servant: but I am slow of speech, and of a slow tongue." Realizing this weakness and the importance of speaking in his new appointment, Moses wasn't confident about fulfilling God's request. God then responded to Moses with words of assurance and reminded him that He was the Maker of man and He therefore knew all about Moses' speech and He would teach him what to say (Exodus 4:12).

Despite all God said, Moses did not want to speak to the people. Yet, God was adamant about using Moses to deliver His people. So in order to appease Moses, God allowed Aaron, Moses' brother, to be the spokesperson. God's directive to Moses was that Aaron should speak only the words Moses told him to say, which, by the way, would be the words God would speak to Moses (Exodus 4:13–17).

Sometimes assistance is needed from others in order for us to accomplish God's will. This happened with Moses, and it frequently happens with caregivers. Oftentimes, caregivers cannot or will not adequately state their needs. When this happens, the coordinator will be in place to be the voice of the caregiver.

Yes, indeed, the role of the caregiver coordinator is biblical!

# Chapter 13
## The Coordinator's Oath of Responsibility

THE CAREGIVER COORDINATOR has been called alongside the caregiver to be as Aaron was to Moses—a spokesperson. Operating in the capacity of a spokesperson, the coordinator's role is to be the voice of the caregiver in an effort to ease the caregiver's responsibilities while caring for the patient. By no means does this appointment imply that the spokesperson must take control and handle matters outside of the caregiver's wishes. The role of the caregiver's coordinator is to respond according to the instructions provided by the caregiver.

In absence of the caregiver, situations should be handled the way that God would. That is to say, whatever Jesus would do, then that's what the coordinator must do as well. The coordinator must carry out this ministry the way the caregiver desires; any other way is not acceptable.

# Chapter 14
## Should Family Members be Appointed as Coordinators?

IN SOME CASES, a close family member is ready to step in and assume the role of coordinator. Yet, this may not always be the ideal appointment for a family member. Consider this: when a family is already experiencing a crisis, all members are affected to some degree. If having a family member be the coordinator makes matters worse, then that family appointee could lose focus and not be able to function adequately. Every situation is unique, so choose what is best for the circumstances at hand.

# Chapter 15
## Who Should be Appointed as Coordinator?

THE COORDINATOR'S POSITION is not for the person who has demonstrated little or no respect for other people's privacy. Certainly no one who is a known gossiper should be considered as a coordinator. (This person has problems of his or her own that need to be resolved prior to his or her assisting others!) There are also other categories of people who would not make good coordinators but would perhaps work perfectly in other areas. If this is the case, find those areas and let those people use their godly-inspired gifts to help the patient and the caregiver. Jesus told His disciples in Mark 9:40, "For he that is not against us is on our part."

# Chapter 16
## Who Will Help Mobile Families to Receive Assistance?

**W**E NOW LIVE in communities that consist of families of which many are mobile. This means that many people, especially military families, are far removed from relatives and friends. When considering a coordinator for military families, someone who understands their world would be the best choice. In cases where there is no church membership, the local church should step up and offer services to families who are facing a crisis and/or need assistance. What better way for kingdom people to show the love of God than to help a stranger in need?

> Then shall the King say unto them on his right hand, Come, ye blessed of my Father, inherit the kingdom prepared for you from the foundation of the world: For I was an hungred, and ye gave me meat: I was thirsty, and ye gave me drink: I was a stranger, and ye took me in: Naked, and ye clothed me: I was sick, and ye visited me: I was in prison, and ye came unto me. Then shall the righteous answer him, saying, Lord, when saw we thee an hungred, and fed thee? or thirsty, and gave thee drink? When saw we thee a stranger, and took thee in? or naked, and clothed thee? Or when saw we thee sick, or in prison, and came unto thee? And the King shall answer and say unto them, Verily I say unto you, Inasmuch as ye have done it unto one of the least of these my brethren, ye have done it unto me.
> —Matt. 25:34–40

# Chapter 17
## Should an Alternate Coordinator be Appointed?

THE KEY TO the successful administration of this ministry is in knowing both the severity of the crisis and the family's needs. If the crisis is severe, it may be wise to appoint an alternate coordinator at the very beginning. However, an alternate may not be needed; therefore, he or she may never fully function in this capacity. What circumstances would necessitate the alternate's assuming the role of the primary coordinator should be clearly established. Again, family needs are the focus.

While one primary coordinator is a necessity, several helpers also could be appointed. For example, one helper could be someone at the patient's and/or caregiver's place of employment, another could be a person at church, and still another could be assigned to handle all communication matters.

With my husband's medical situation, I primarily kept one person at the military base, where he was employed, abreast of his condition. This person communicated updates and my requests/needs to others at the base. This type of assignment can be done for as many areas that need coverage: work, church, clubs/organizations, schools, etc. (See chapter 38 for information regarding updating school teachers when children are affected.)

# Chapter 18
# Managing Negative Responses

WITH EVERY MINISTRY, problems will arise. Therefore, the coordinator must be prepared for whatever problems may surface, including negative responds from family members and friends. Some people may even criticize, second guess, or challenge decisions made by the caregiver and/or coordinator. This could be Satan's response to something positive. Realize from the beginning that Satan's main purpose is to tear down what God is sustaining. For this reason, do not take attacks personally. This is just one of the reasons why at least one person needs to be appointed to pray daily for the patient, caregiver, caregiver's coordinator, and others. (See chapter 23.)

The coordinator can help alleviate Satan's impact by assuring inquirers that the caregiver's instructions are being followed. Realize, too, that the coordinator is their perceived threat because this is the person who is preventing them from getting close to the patient and/or caregiver. Keep in mind that they probably just want to express their concern in their own special way. They do not purposely intend to harm anyone by thinking only of themselves and their desires.

## Managing Negative Responses

Soliciting suggestions from these inquirers that can then be communicated to the caregiver also may help to ease the tension. And still another way to lessen the negative response of others is to always let whatever is done be sanctioned by the caregiver beforehand—not afterward! Communication is a valuable tool. Use it!

# Chapter 19
# Caregiver's Basic Instructions to the Coordinator

IN THE EVENT that prior planning is possible, a list of dos and don'ts for the caregiver coordinator should be established. If feasible, both the caregiver and patient should contribute to this list. Accomplishing this in advance will alleviate many difficult moments and provide the greatest understanding among family members and friends. However, in emergencies, when advanced planning is not possible, all decisions that are made become a matter of necessity. When advanced planning *is* possible, be sure to take advantage of this precious opportunity.

Again, let me assure you, this assistance is not expected to last indefinitely! It is only necessary until the situation is stabilized and becomes manageable for the caregiver. In some cases, assistance will be needed for a longer period, but it will not be as intense as when the need first arose.

# Chapter 20
# Establishing Communication Lists

THE PURPOSE OF establishing a notification list is to keep those who have a genuine concern about the patient and caregiver abreast of what is occurring in their lives. The purpose is not to broadcast their business! Too much information circulating can fall into the hands of the wrong person, i.e. burglars and other criminals. So be very careful about who has access to the information and who is being notified.

# Chapter 21
## Communication: The Inner Circle

THE COMMUNICATION PROTOCOL should be established first. The caregiver, not the coordinator, should establish separate lists of people and the order in which they are to be notified of events/updates regarding the patient. The caregiver should start out first by designating an inner circle, those whom he or she will be responsible for contacting.

My primary inner circle consisted of our children, my mother-in-law, our pastor, and my husband's temporary primary care doctor. Our youngest child lived with us, so he was the first to *see* the effects of my husband's illness. I look back now and realize that I did not communicate with him as I should have. I allowed his age, fifteen, and the fact that he was in the home, to prevent me from sharing as much as I should have. I actually shared more information with his older sister and brother than I did with him. The other two children were informed mainly by telephone, as were my mother-in law and our pastor.

Whenever conditions worsened, which seemed quite often at first, I would apprise my husband's doctor so that she was aware of the medical problems, could keep the referral order for care open, and would be willing to provide other referrals when necessary. (This doctor was the person who ordered the appropriate tests that

## Communication: The Inner Circle

resulted in the brain tumor being discovered. Once the tumor was diagnosed, referral was made to a neurologist at another hospital, who assumed responsibility for his care. Requests for travel for me as well as for my husband also were procured through this doctor.) After this inner circle was informed, then notification to others followed.

# Chapter 22
## Other Communication Lists

I HAD THREE layers of my communication circle—my inner circle (we already talked about them in the previous chapter); a circle that consisted primarily of family members and friends, most of whom I knew did not have e-mail; and then a very broad circle that consisted of those to whom I provided updates via e-mail. (See chapter 24 for more on this mode of communication.) I also provided brief updates for everyone who inquired via telephone, in the community, in the workplace, etc.

Communicating updates to everyone who wanted to be notified of my husband's condition was very exhausting for me. This was due in part to the size of my husband's and my families. We both come from very large families, and we have so many friends who love us! Praise God! Nevertheless, having to voice my husband's condition to every person I did communicate with was like reliving a traumatic event with every telling of the details surrounding his medical condition. While dealing with the actuality of a situation helps to provide healing, having to retell the events beyond the therapeutic point is not. I agree that testimonies should be shared with others; however, the appropriate time for a testimony is when it helps the giver and the receiver.

Other Communication Lists

Communicating with others is one area in which a coordinator can help the most. A coordinator or helper can be the voice for the caregiver, providing as little or as much information to others as the caregiver sanctions.

# Chapter 23
## Appointing Prayer Warriors

UNDERGIRD THIS MINISTRY with prayer. A situation not covered in prayer is a situation that is open for Satan to destroy. Therefore, designate someone or solicit volunteers to pray daily for those directly affected by the crisis. The list of those who are being prayed for should include the patient, caregiver, other family members, and the coordinator. These individual names should be called out in prayer every day! Others who need prayer, whose names may not be known, are the doctors, nurses, other medical staff members, and all those who will partner with the coordinator to render assistance.

# Chapter 24
# Communicating via the Internet (Web sites) or E-mail

THE COORDINATOR SHOULD always use the approved communication list when notifying others of updates on the patient's situation. The coordinator also should be made aware of those whom the caregiver will contact directly. Those on the "inner circle" list *never* should be contacted by the coordinator unless the caregiver gives permission. Those on this list are people whom the caregiver and patient want to communicate with directly, so respect their wishes. It has nothing to do with the coordinator not being able to communicate with them. It is a matter of courtesy.

The coordinator always needs to get the caregiver's approval of the information that will be sent out to others. When he or she is sending an e-mail, a subject line should be included, such as: "Update on **(provide name of sick person)** as of **(provide date)**." If possible, he or she should include in the body of the e-mail when the reader can expect to receive a follow-up message. For example, if an MRI or other critical tests are pending, it should be noted in the e-mail that an update will be sent as soon as test results are made available. Only necessary information needs to be communicated; keep the communication to a minimum! For a gauge, weekly is good, but when a patient's condition changes dramatically, information should be communicated more regularly.

The coordinator should keep in mind that many people have a genuine concern, so if there are no changes, he or she can simply post a message each week stating that fact.

Another thing that the coordinator must remember is that releasing information about the patient and caregiver being away from home could fall into the hands of predators. Empty houses are a target for criminals, so he or she needs to be very careful about what information is shared and with whom.

This type of communication will be less frequent as the crisis diminishes and as the caregiver is able to assume this responsibility. Remember, this responsibility will not last forever.

# Chapter 25
# Using Facebook as a Means of Communication

THE COORDINATOR MAY need to explain to the patient and caregiver the different means of communication that are available. Whether or not to use Facebook or some other mode of communication is a decision that the patient and/or caregiver should make. Once this is done, the coordinator should always use that preferred method. Remember, the coordinator is in place to assist the caregiver by responding to his or her requests.

I used e-mail to communicate with others. Yet, there are other options that are user friendly and offer more privacy. (For more information, read the next chapter.)

# Chapter 26
## Alternative Care Pages: Free Web sites

NUMEROUS FREE WEB sites, such as http://www.caringbridge.org/, are available that allow for patient information to be posted. This is by far the easiest way to keep those who have computers abreast of the patient's condition, because once the information is posted, it can be accessed twenty-four hours a day! Also, a site such as this has an aroma of respect and sensitivity that patients need.

Some hospitals offer free Web sites that can be used to communicate updates about patients. Be sure to check with the hospital in advance for this service.

In situations where someone besides the caregiver is maintaining this site, information should always be pre-approved by the caregiver. Again, care should always be taken when releasing information.

## Chapter 27

# Can Men Function as Coordinators?

MALES OR FEMALES can function in the role of caregiver coordinator. The gender of the coordinator is not a major concern. The main requirement is that the person is someone who can handle the organizing of care. In situations where the caregiver is a female, a female may function best as coordinator, and vice versa. This way people of the same sex are communicating with one another and any problems of infidelity that possibly may occur can be minimized.

If men prefer not to function in the role of a coordinator, that is perfectly acceptable. Caring, strong men are always needed to move furniture, help lift a fallen patient, unclog sinks, and do many other tasks, so they should not feel they have nothing to contribute to this ministry. Men are also great at taking care of outdoor tasks, i.e. washing vehicles, trimming hedges, mowing lawns, etc. Some, like my husband, even love to cook! So when men volunteer their services, let them help.

# Chapter 28
## Sending Flowers to the Patient

IF PEOPLE DESIRE to send flowers, they should be made aware of certain hospital restrictions, i.e. flowers are not allowed in the ICU. In addition, either the patient or caregiver may be allergic to different types of flowers. Without knowing some things in advance, purchasing flowers will end up being a good gesture that benefits no one but the sender. Also, because removal of the flowers may become the responsibility of the family, an additional, unnecessary burden occurs if the patient is transferred to another hospital.

The coordinator also may suggest to those who want to send flowers to wait and not send the flowers to the patient while he or she is in the hospital, but instead, encourage them to send a card. Inside the card, they can enclose a self-address, stamped postcard with a note on it that says, "Please send my flowers!" This way, when the patient's condition has stabilized or when he or she has returned home, the card can be mailed back to the person who wanted to give the flowers. Upon receipt of the postcard, the giver of the flowers can arrange to have the flowers delivered when they will be most appreciated.

The coordinator should not be hesitant about maybe even suggesting an artificial flower arrangement, if this is the preference of the patient or caregiver. Depending on the time

## Sending Flowers to the Patient

of the year, another suggestion would be to have the person buy outdoor flowers, then arrange a time when he or she can come to the home for a brief visit to plant the flowers outside in a designated area.

## Chapter 29
## Helping Out-of-Towners to Lend a Helping Hand

COORDINATORS, BE BOLD! Always provide suggestions for different ways in which out-of-towners can contribute if they desire. If a list of needed items is not established, most people will resort to sending flowers. (See chapter 28.) There is nothing wrong with this gesture, but kindness can be extended in so many different and useful ways. Below is a brief list. Suggest the purchaser give:

- Gift cards to CVS, Wal-mart, Walgreens, or other similar stores where prescriptions can be filled and miscellaneous items can be purchased.
- New clothing items—sometimes new items will be needed. Not all patients lose weight, some gain due to steroids and/or other medicines.
- One hour of cleaning service for the home. (Check out companies in advance. The patient or caregiver may already use a company on special occasions.)
- Money! It is always needed and gladly accepted. (The cost of medicine, even the co-pay, is outrageous. The gas needed to travel back and forth to the hospital can get to be very costly. If the patient was employed, then an income

probably is not being generated. Additionally, depending on the illness, sick leave and/or long- or short-term disability could be depleted prior to when the patient can return to work. Also, if the caregiver is employed, he or she is missing days from work; therefore, no income is being generated, and the availability of sick leave could be a problem for him or her too.) Very few people are in a position where money is not needed, so when a person is in doubt as to what to send, send money!

Patients' and caregivers' needs vary from situation to situation. Some cases are more severe than others, so the coordinator should be aware of their immediate needs in order to guide the person who wants to give to the area where help is most needed.

## Chapter 30
## Other Suggestions for Out-of-Towners

CREATE A LIST of needs that will work for everyone involved—the patient, caregiver, and children (if they are affected directly by the crisis). Listed below are additional suggestions.

- Vehicle maintenance coupons or gift certificates (oil changes, tune-ups, etc.)
- Carwash coupons or gift certificates
- Gas coupons or gift cards
- Stamps (to send thank you cards)
- Lawn care service gift certificates
- Restaurant gift cards (fast food for on-the-go meals)
- Alteration/dry cleaning coupons or gift certificates
- Salon and/or barber shop gift certificates
- Gift cards/certificates to various other useful places

Use the lines below to list other suggestions.

_____
_____
_____
_____

# Chapter 31
## Miscellaneous Services the Patient Will Need at Home

THE CAREGIVER WILL need help in assisting the patient to look his or her best. (When a person looks good, oftentimes he or she feels good—or perhaps, better.) Seek someone from the generated list of partners to take care of the patient's grooming needs. If no one can accommodate this need, consider arranging for the patient's regular barber/beautician to come to the home. Home visits are necessary because normally services on location are very tiring and intrusive. When planning, the coordinator needs to be sure not to subject the patient or the caregiver to an unnecessary service too soon. (This visit also could be the barber/beautician's contribution to the patient and caregiver, so let him or her know in advance why services are needed at home.)

When my mom was nearing the end of her earthly life, her beautician provided services in her home. She did this free of charge, but of course, Mom insisted on paying and tipping! This same beautician also styled Mom's hair for her final viewing. This time her services were provided as a token of love to our family.

Another service that is very helpful is having meals brought to the home of the patient. Arrange for different groups to bring meals to the home already prepared. Have these generous people keep in mind the special diets of both the patient and the caregiver. Refrain from having meals prepared in the home because the kitchen is not familiar to the preparer; therefore, this service could be more of an inconvenience than a help. Besides, when a person is sick, the smell of food being prepared can be nauseating.

In addition to the above, the following services may need to be coordinated with those who are partnering with the coordinator:

- Drivers to take the patient to doctors' visits
- Grocery pickup
- Clean-up inside and outside the home, i.e. lawn maintenance
- Answering the telephone/receiving visitors

Record other services the patient and caregiver may need in the blanks below.

_____
_____
_____
_____
_____
_____
_____
_____
_____
_____
_____
_____

# Chapter 32
## Types of Services the Patient Does Not Need!

NEITHER CAREGIVERS NOR coordinators should feel compelled to accept inadequate services offered by any company. Every company has policies and standards they must follow; therefore, if the service being given is not what was advertised or as expected, cancel the service and report the company. Life for the patient and caregiver is stressful enough, so companies that are not sensitive to the needs of the sick should not be allowed to continue operating in a non-caring manner.

I was moved by God to eliminate a service my husband was receiving that was not adequate. I had to; otherwise, their lack of performance and insensitivity to our needs would have highly affected our sanity and my husband's care.

To give you a general idea of what we encountered, I share the following story. For a very short time, a local company contracted by the military provided home healthcare to my husband. With this service, we encountered many obstacles because the services were very limited and not as useful as advertised. There was no direct access to a physician. In fact, we were told the best they could do was to call in our situation and wait for a response from someone who would then relay the information to the on-call doctor. (Although my husband's doctor was located in another city, I had direct access to either him or a team member who assisted with the surgery. I always talked directly to a doctor!)

Another area of concern was the providers with this company were constantly late. Even on the day of the initial intake, the nurse was over an hour late! Depending on the level of sickness of a patient, this may not be a concern. However, in our situation, it was a tremendous concern. My husband's nap, eating, and taking medicine were all centered on the provider's arriving at the appointed time. Tardiness threw off our entire schedule!

Loss of data or their not entering my husband's medical information was another concern. Because the information was not entered into the system (thus making it available to everyone who needed to view the required information) every person who visited our home would ask the same questions upon arrival. On several occasions, I watched my husband repeatedly being drilled for the same information until my heart could not take it any longer. I wanted to give the information myself and waited several times for the nurse to turn to me to get it, but this never happened.

Ultimately, this service was more of a nuisance than a help, so I contacted the appropriate office and explained the situation to them. Of course, this meant I was now alone again on this journey, but I felt there was no need for a service of this sort to continue.

If something of this nature happens to you, consider reporting the agency so that the company can correct their way of providing service. This reporting is done so that the next person will not have to endure receiving inadequate service. Help is needed, but not on a hit-and-miss basis. Consistent care is needed for any situation.

# Chapter 33
## The Patient and Caregiver's New Way of Life

THE COORDINATOR CAN be helpful in not allowing others to impose on either the caregiver or the patient by asking duties of either before both have given their consent to resume normal activities. Realize that sometimes this consent is never given. Keep in mind, the purpose of this book is to provide guidance for those whose medical conditions warrant the services of a caregiver and a coordinator to assist the caregiver. This means the condition is serious. Serious conditions do not heal overnight. Therefore, everyone should give patients and their caregivers the time needed to heal, as well as the time needed to adjust to a new way of life.

Nearly three years have passed since my husband's initial surgery, and we are still adjusting to our new limitations! While we realize that our lives will never be the same as they were prior to the surgery, family and friends see the same frame on the outside, and some may assume that things are the same as they were before. Unfortunately, when a major surgery has taken place, or if a patient is dealing with a life-threatening illness, the condition of the body on the inside undergoes continuous changes. The mental state is also affected. For example, before a medical crisis, the patient and/or caregiver may have been known to be pleasant and even-tempered, but now he or she always seem to be agitated, angry, or even depressed. (If this occurs, the treating physician should be informed of this new illness and family members should be sympathetic and willing to assist in any way possible.)

My husband's surgery had the impact of an earthquake hitting our lives. As a result, my husband no longer can perform some duties as he did in the past. Because of this, many responsibilities shifted to me. Foster, our youngest son, also acquired some new responsibilities—mainly, he got permanent lawn duty! Some other things in our lives were completely eliminated; they were buried in the vault caused by the massive earthquake. We simply cannot function as we once did, which also means that some of our pleasurable activities are now gone.

Yet, as it is with any long-term illness, our focus and response to life is refined. We no longer sweat the small stuff. We do what we can, when we can. And whatever we do, we do it with great joy, knowing that God is pleased with the little that we are doing!

## Chapter 34
## When Should Hospice be Considered?

HOSPICE? EVEN THE word "hospice" is hard for some people to say. When this service is needed, someone from the hospital will make the suggestion to the family. If the suggestion is made, the coordinator is in a position to gently encourage the caregiver, if he or she is not already receptive to the referral. Hospice personnel are trained to take some of the burden off the caregiver by providing a variety of services.

My personal experience with hospice occurred many years ago, during my Mom's illness. During those very difficult days, hospice was in place to assist with our family's needs. Their assistance made it possible for Mom to be at home as she requested, and it relieved the family of many minor tasks. Hospice gave us the precious time we wanted to spend with Mom before she was taken up to heaven.

# Chapter 35
## Give the Caregiver Plenty of Breaks!

THE MOST APPROPRIATE time to help is when people are hurting and are in need. The purpose of this ministry is to have a coordinator assist in putting in place outside support that will help to ease the responsibilities of the caregiver. This support mechanism gives an opportunity for the caregiver to have the distance he or she needs from the situation. Therefore, it is important for the coordinator to be available so that the caregiver will have no excuse for not taking time for him or herself. Even in the absence of a coordinator to assist with care giving, if every person who reads this book will help someone they know, a tremendous burden will be lifted from the caregiver's shoulders.

If I had to give myself a grade in this area, then I must be honest with you and let you know that as a caregiver, I very rarely distanced myself from the patient; therefore, I made an F! This is the hardest area I had to cope with. Guilt enslaved me into thinking that every time I took time for myself, I was being selfish. Every time I was separated from my husband, other than for work or other necessary functions, I felt guilty. Although I knew I needed time for myself, actually taking the time was extremely difficult.

On one occasion, when my husband was hospitalized locally, the doctors decided it was best for him to be transferred to the city where his surgery was performed. Since our youngest child was in school, I made the decision to stay behind to take care of his needs. Once the transfer took place, I informed my husband's temporary primary care doctor at the local base. After I finished dialoging about my husband, the doctor then turned her focus to me. She asked me, "How are you doing?" Her soft, caring words opened up a fountain I did not know was welling up inside of me. My face felt as if I had been doused with a bucket of water. For a moment or two, I was speechless. It was truly refreshing to know that she was genuinely concerned about me.

The doctor then gave me the best advice needed for our situation. She told me that while my husband was in another city to not worry about him because he was being taken care of by specialists—some of the best doctors in the country. According to her, what I needed to do was to focus on me, to take care of my needs. I was told not to engage in any cleaning or other unnecessary tasks. She told me to rest, to use this time to refresh myself. We've all heard the words of wisdom given to new mothers—to sleep when the baby sleeps!—well I did exactly what the doctor ordered, so by the time I needed to resume my hands-on caregiving, I was rejuvenated.

Yet, the refreshing didn't last long! Perhaps it was because the illness continued well past the time I expected it to last. It got to the point where I often felt guilty about being at work all day. However, I frequently tried to do something pleasurable for myself. On one occasion, after arriving home from work, I quickly changed into my gym clothes. As I was headed out of the house to drive to the gym, tears started to coat my eyes. As I traveled the short distance from home to the gym, I kept wanting to turn around and go back home. Then, once I arrived at the gym and began to walk on the track, I literally stopped in the middle of exercising to go back home. However, I did not go. I completed my forty-five minute workout, but I struggled. My workout wasn't as refreshing as it should have been.

I also recall using my lunch hour, along with an hour of leave, to pick up lunch and go home to check on my husband. After the crisis was over, I mentioned to a friend that this was one area where help from others was desperately needed. In fact, this family friend had actually taken lunch to my husband and kept him company on one occasion. This kind gesture enabled me to use my lunch break for myself that day.

Blinded by my own guilt and anxiety, all I saw was the need to go home in order to break the monotony my husband was experiencing from being home alone throughout the day. Anybody could have met that need! It wasn't until much later that I realized my own needs and began to take time for myself without feeling guilty.

I've learned so much from my husband's illness. That's why I'm sharing my mistakes in this book so that others will not make the same mistakes I did! I do not want any caregiver to travel the same path I traveled. My desire for them is that they will have someone to partner with them as they go through a difficult time in their lives. You can help a caregiver avoid some of the pitfalls I encountered, by partnering with them.

Below are a few activities that can be recommended to a caregiver to help him or her get some distance from the patient for a brief period.

- Reading a book
- Working out in a gym
- Shopping
- Walking in the park
- Visiting a friend
- Participating in a sporting event
- Having lunch or dinner with friends

As other activities come to mind, add them to the list.

_____

_____

_____

Give the Caregiver Plenty of Breaks!

# Chapter 36
## Encourage the Caregiver to Seek Support from Other Caregivers

ONE UNIQUE THING about an illness is that it isolates the patient and the caregiver from the rest of the world. For this reason, and many others, the caregiver should be encouraged to connect with others who have or have had similar experiences. There are so many people in the world who are hurting and need to find comfort in a support group; they just do not know where to go.

About six months after my husband's surgery, I sought to find a local brain tumor support group in my area by asking friends who were in the medical profession. These friends told me repeatedly that the only services available were those offered through formal counseling. At this point, I solicited help from my husband's doctors. However, no one was able to locate a support group in my area. This is when I ventured out on my own to locate one. With the aid of the Internet, in September of 2009, nearly two years after the initial surgery, I found two support groups that were located about 140 miles away, in another state. I contacted the coordinator of one group and expressed our desire to attend. We have been attending ever since.

By attending the support group sessions on a regular basis, we both have been helped beyond measure. My husband has been able

## Encourage the Caregiver to Seek Support from Other Caregivers

to understand more about his illness from others in the group. He has a better understanding of his limitations and has become quite the counselor himself! As a caregiver, I am able to understand how my husband's condition affects him, me, and the entire family, as well as how to respond to his needs and my own. I also have learned that guilt is a common emotion felt by many caregivers, but that guilt should not paralyze us.

Coping with an illness is extremely difficult when a person does not understand the mechanisms of the illness. Yet when others provide insight, the journey is more pleasurable and manageable. Two of our children, Jacinta and Foster, have also attended the support group meetings.

Since we have been attending this support group, a support group for children has been established. There has been an overwhelming need for this ministry because children need to learn how to cope as well.

For those who cannot find a support group in the immediate area, the *National Family Caregivers Association* has a Web site especially designed to address the needs of caregivers. This site, http://www.nfcacares.org, contains a variety of information, but most importantly, it provides a mechanism for caregivers to communicate with one another. Just knowing that at least one person cares can make all the difference in the world to a caregiver who has reached a point of despondency.

# Chapter 37
# Calling Partners/Agencies for Assistance

WHEN IN NEED, the coordinator should insist that the caregiver call for help. Also, he or she should remember to utilize the list of family members and friends who indicated they can respond at a moment's notice.

I did not have a call list, so when I needed to take my husband to the Emergency Room around midnight on a school night, with no one in the home to stay with our son, I had a problem. I had no biological family in the area to call, so because of my experience, I implore you, caregiver or coordinator, to make a list of individuals who are willing to assist in times of a crisis!

When utilizing the call-in service of electric and gas companies, care should be taken to alert the service providers that a seriously-ill person resides in the household. Companies will normally place these work orders in a higher category, thereby reducing the response time to the home.

A list of local agencies who can lend a helping hand should also be created. For example, the fire department can assist when the patient falls and is too heavy for any available person to lift. (I have learned this happens quite often!) When needed, call their non-emergency number, and they normally will respond right away.

Calling Partners/Agencies for Assistance

Record the names of other agencies and their telephone numbers in the blanks on the following page. This list should be updated as the patient's medical needs change.

Telephone numbers of agencies to call for immediate assistance:

_____
_____
_____
_____
_____
_____
_____
_____
_____
_____
_____
_____
_____
_____
_____
_____
_____
_____

# Chapter 38
## Caring for the Children in the Family

UP TO NOW, the primary focus has been on the patient and the caregiver. However, we must remember that children also have needs. They should not be overlooked! While the caregiver is directly responsible for the children, the coordinator can help by reminding the caregiver of matters related to the children that need addressing.

One very important matter is school. The parent/guardian should make every effort possible to inform their children's teachers of a family emergency. While it is true that children may not know everything related to the crisis, they do recognize that things are different. Many children will show a behavior change when a family is dealing with a crisis. Alerting teachers to this crisis will help them to be of assistance to the children.

When my husband was in the military and was out of the country on a temporary assignment, I informed every one of my children's teachers, including those at the daycare center where our youngest child attended. Because the daycare staff knew of the absence of the child's father, when he experienced days when he cried for apparently no reason at all, the staff understood the reason for the tears and could comfort him appropriately.

## Caring for the Children in the Family

The parent/guardian should keep teachers abreast of a family crisis and inform them if another person also will be communicating updates to them in cases where the parent/guardian cannot. In addition, the parent/guardian should always ensure the necessary forms that will allow a designated person to pick up their children from school are completed.

I communicated with our son's high school teachers via e-mail. Every teacher responded with his or her willingness to assist because they understood that what we were experiencing as a family could affect our child's performance in school. The names we had on the list of people to pick him up from school were sufficient, so I did not need to visit the school to take care of this matter.

Learning to communicate with the children about the crisis is also important. The caregiver may be so absorbed by other duties that he or she neglects to or simply does not know how to communicate the crisis to the children. Do not just assume they know what is occurring. Allow them to express themselves in their own ways. Some do this best by drawing or acting out their emotions.

Someone also should be designated to stay overnight in the children's home if necessary. Since frequent unannounced trips to the hospital are common for patients who are critical, having this matter taken care of in advance will bring comfort to the caregiver and security to the children.

When needed, a designated driver should be in place to transport the children of the caregiver to church, school, extracurricular activities, the hospital, shopping for necessities, etc. Every family's needs are different, so as other places come to mind, add them to the list.

_____

_____

_____

_____

One of my biggest regrets in regards to my children's needs was not having someone in place to continue taking our son, Foster, to football games. Foster was in the ninth grade, but because he traveled with the varsity football team up to the time when his dad had surgery, he was considered a member of the team. This membership was extremely important, because his team, the Lowndes County Vikings, won the state championship that year. Had Foster continued traveling with the team, he would have received a ring and varsity athlete's jacket, just like every other team member did. Even today, when I think about this event, my heart aches and I feel guilty for not coordinating with someone to take Foster to the few remaining games of the season.

Now, as we approach Foster's last year in high school, I pray this will be another championship year for the Vikings. This request may sound selfish to some, but so be it. My heart's desire is for my child to receive in 2010 what he was deprived of because of my oversight in 2007.

# Chapter 39
# Arrange Fun Time for the Children— Give Them a Break!

JUST LIKE THE caregiver needs distance, children need the same! With the parent(s) permission, the children should be treated to a day at the park, eating out, shopping, skating, etc. If money is not an obstacle, a partner may even want to consider indulging them in their favorite activity.

Many organizations recognize the need for children to have fun. This need is met by offering free passes to families who either have a terminally ill parent or child. One such organization is *Memories of Love*. Please use the following Web site to find out more information, http://www.memoriesoflove.org/. *Wishing Grant Organization* provides a Web site, http://www.familyvillage.wisc.edu/general/wish-grant-orgs.html, which includes numerous names of organizations that provide this same type of service. The coordinator or partner can visit the site and choose the place that is best for the family.

# Chapter 40
## Family Matters

IN CHAPTER 33, I mentioned the word "refined" as it applies to the new life my family now has. Along with the spiritual and emotional healing, physical healing in our lives had to occur. God assisted in that healing by pruning many activities from our lives. In our season of doing, we did what was required of us (Ecclesiastes 3:1). Now, we are not physically able to endure those same activities. Therefore, the things that we do are fewer in number, but they have a greater meaning to us. We fully understand that it is not the quantity that matters; it's the quality. Above all things, it is the condition of the servant's heart.

Obtaining a balance took time, and it was painful, but now that we have it, our lives are continuously being enriched. It is as though God took us to another spiritual level in our understanding of who He is. Although this change wasn't pleasant and at times was very painful, we find comfort in the fact that God was glorified. Therefore, our change, from beginning to end, has been worth every teardrop that fell from our eyes.

# Conclusion

Jesus said unto him, Thou shalt love the Lord thy God with all thy heart, and with all thy soul, and with all thy mind. This is the first and great commandment. And the second is like unto it, Thou shalt love thy neighbor as thyself. On these two commandments hang all the law and the prophets.

—Matt. 22:37–40

Therefore all things whatsoever ye would that men should do to you, do ye even so to them: for this is the law and the prophets.

—Matt. 7:12

CARE GIVING IS like an all-consuming fire, reaching into the depths of a person's physical, mental, emotional, and spiritual state. It leaves scars in every area of a person's life: religious, professional, social, personal, financial, etc. To sum up the reality about care giving, *it is very stressful!* Yet, some of the stress can be minimized, even eliminated, if concerned, caring people will partner with the caregiver during his or her time of need.

The Word of God, in 2 Corinthians 1:3–4 tells us that we are comforted to comfort others. This means that we must take what we have learned and help others. Because I am now a caregiver, I have a greater understanding of the need for a ministry that focuses on the needs of caregivers. This is why I am advocating for partners to assist us.

In this book are lists containing simple suggestions to help establish this ministry and ideas on how people (family, friends, co-workers, etc.) can partner with a caregiver. You should have discovered ways to:

- Help the caregiver.
- Help the caregiver coordinator understand his or her role.
- Help family and friends (concerned loved ones) understand the dynamics of this ministry.
- Help family and friends become participants in this ministry.
- Help families, churches, work groups, and/or community groups establish a caregiver support ministry. (This ministry can be established amongst any network of people who are available and willing to help meet the needs of the patient and caregiver.)

Beloved, you, and many more like you, are needed to partner with caregivers. If every concerned person who reads this book will help a caregiver by simply lending a helping hand in one or more of the areas mentioned, burdens will be lifted and life will be more pleasurable for all involved in this neighborly ministry of love. I know you might be a little hesitant and concerned about partnering with caregivers, but I implore you to step out in faith and just allow God to use you in whatever capacity He desires. Through your obedience, healings will transpire.

Someone somewhere needs your help. The question is, will you respond?

—Verna

# About the Author

**Verna Foster Harvey** is a teacher who has a heart for God's people. For over fifteen years, she has been actively studying and passionately teaching others about God, either one-on-one or in a group setting. The messages she teaches are entwined with current events and accompanied by many practical applications, helping to facilitate learning for all age groups. Because of Verna's belief in openness, she frequently shares episodes from her life with the listening audience.

Valdosta, Georgia, is home for Verna and Lenon, her husband of over thirty years. They have three children, a daughter-in-law, three grandchildren, and a godson. Their youngest child, Foster, a high school student, resides with them. The Harveys are active members of Crossroads Baptist Church in the city in which they live.

# Verna's Books

Please visit Verna's Web page at http://www.livingtogive.org to inquire about her books:

*Partnering with Caregivers: Learn How to Help Those Who Help Others* (2010)

*The Blessedness of Waiting on God: How to Deal with the Stress of Holding Patterns* (2007)

*Growing God's Way: The Pathway from Salvation to Heaven is Filled with Growing Pains!* (2004)

While visiting Verna's Web page, please click on the "Sign up for weekly devotional" box to start receiving her devotional entitled: "Refreshing Moments with God."

## Contacting the Author

Use the e-mail address*,
verna@livingtogive.org,
to inquire about speaking events
or to schedule a book read or book signing.

*The above e-mail address may also be used to send comments about her books or to post comments at the various Web sites where her books are sold.

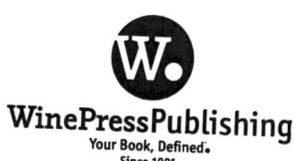

**WinePressPublishing**
Your Book, Defined.
Since 1991.

To order additional copies of this book call:
1-877-421-READ (7323)
or please visit our website at
www.WinePressbooks.com

If you enjoyed this quality custom-published book,
drop by our website for more books and information.

www.winepresspublishing.com
"Your partner in custom publishing."

CPSIA information can be obtained at www.ICGtesting.com
Printed in the USA
LVOW07s1111141213

365315LV00005B/1430/P